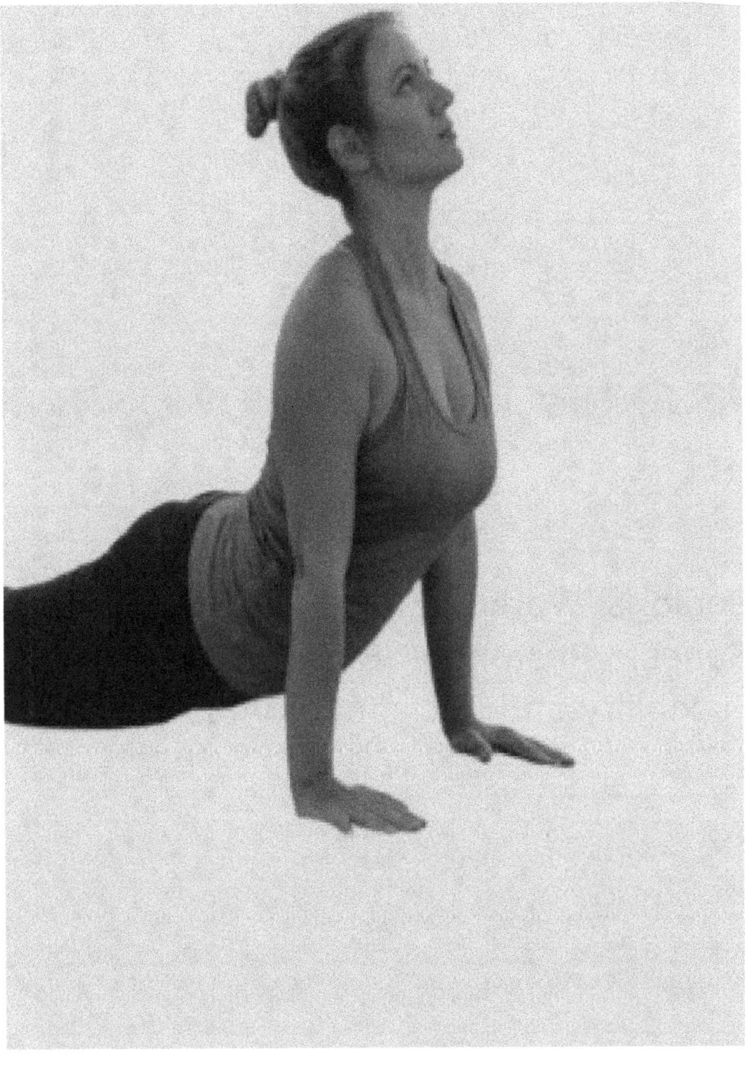

40 EXERCISES FOR STRONGER BONES

Senior's Workout for Building Stronger Bones, Restoring Balance, Improving Flexibility and Reclaiming Vitality.

PAUL KELVIN

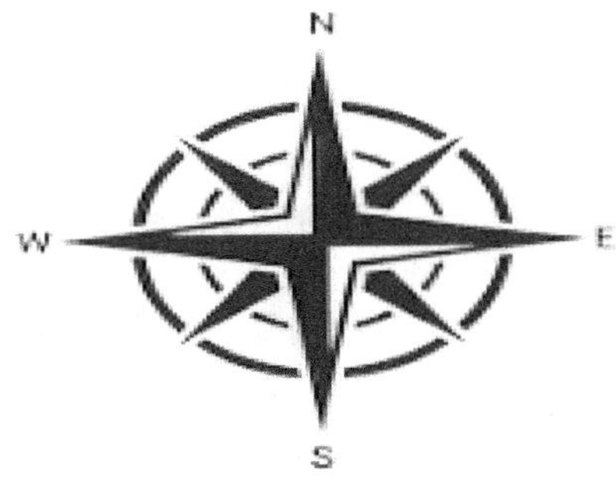

TABLE OF CONTENTS

INTRODUCTION:....................**10**

CHAPTER 1: OSTEOPOROSIS SYMPTOMS, CAUSES, CURE AND PREVENTION **12**

SYMPTOMS OF OSTEOPOROSIS:....15

CAUSES OF OSTEOPOROSIS: 17

DISEASES OR ILLNESSES THAT CAN CAUSE OSTEOPOROSIS:................19

HOW TO MANAGE OR TREAT OSTEOPOROSIS: 21

OSTEOPOROSIS MEDICATION: 23

HOW TO PREVENT OR LOWER THE RISK OF OSTEOPOROSIS: 24

CHAPTER 2: EXERCISES TO IMPROVE BONE DENSITY AND FALL PREVENTION 26

FOOT STOMPS EXERCISE: 27

SHOULDER RAISES EXERCISE:.......29

BICEP CURL EXERCISE: 30

HAMSTRING CURL: 31

SQUATS EXERCISE: 32

LEG RAISES WITH THE HIPS: 33

SINGLE LEG STAND: 34

BALL SIT: 35

CHAPTER 3: SPINE STRENGTHENING EXERCISES FOR OSTEOPOROSIS 36

STANDING POSTURE ALIGNMENT: ..37

ABDOMINAL STRETCHING IN MANEUVER:..........38

TAI CHI (THE GATHERING OF CHI): 40

ISOMETRIC THORACIC EXTENSION WHILE STANDING UP AGAINST A WALL: 42

STANDING HORIZONTALLY SHOULDER ABDUCTION WITH RESISTANCE BAND: 44

SCAPULAR RETRACTION COMBINED WITH PRONE THORACIC EXTENSION: 45

PRESSING THE NECK TOWARDS A RESISTANCE: 47

CHEST LIFTS: 48

SPINE STRENGTHENING EXERCISE: 49

CHAPTER 4: OSTEOPOROSIS STRETCHES TO STRENGTHEN THE SHOULDER, NECK AND UPPER SPINE...................50

STRENGTHENING OF THE EXTENSOR MUSCLES: 51

STRENGTHENING THE CALF 52

ACROSS-THE-CHEST STRETCH: 53

SPINAL ROLLS AND EAGLE ARMS: .55

TWIST IN A CHAIR: 56

SHOULDERS CIRCLE: 58

INFANT POSE: 58

PUT THE NEEDLE IN THE THREAD EXERCISE: 59

DOORWAY SHOULDER WORKOUT: .60

DOG POSE DOWNWARD: 61

RELEASE OF THE NECK EXERCISE: .62

CHAPTER 5: OSTEOPOROSIS STRETCHES FOR STRENGTH AND FULL BODY BALANCE 64

CHAIR SQUAT: 64

CHAIR CALF RAISES EXERCISE: 66

LEG SWING BALANCE EXERCISE: ...66

BICEP CURLS USING RESISTANCE BANDS:................................68

TRUNK ROTATION EXERCISE: 69

LYING LEG DROPS EXERCISE: 70

CORE-STRENGTHENING EXERCISE: 71

CHAPTER 6: PILATES STRETCHES TO IMPROVE FLEXIBILITY 73

HIP STRENGTHENING STRETCH: 73

BRIDGE EXERCISE:.......................75

SIDEKICK PILATE: 76

SWAN DIVE PILATE: 78

BIRD DOG PILATE: 79

INTRODUCTION:

With the help of **"40 Exercises for Stronger Bones,"** you will learn how exercises may effectively fight osteoporosis which usually affects seniors.

With careful attention to detail, this ground-breaking book offers an extensive and well-selected selection of 40 exercises that specifically target and strengthen bones, reduce the risk of falls, improve flexibility and give your back control over your skeletal health.

Discover the keys to Increasing bone density, improving balance, increasing flexibility and fostering general well-being as you delve into a realm where traditional knowledge and modern research are used.

This book is your reliable path or route to a healthier, more robust version of yourself, regardless of your level of experience engaging in routine exercises.

A path towards optimal bone health awaits you;

Welcome from a world where osteoporosis and exercise are joined together to provide a path for a healthy future. Allow exercise therapeutic effects to lead you on a journey to long-term health.

CHAPTER 1: OSTEOPOROSIS SYMPTOMS, CAUSES, CURE AND PREVENTION

In this book, we are going to focus on one of the bone disorders called osteoporosis, its symptoms, causes, cure and prevention and the simple exercises that may help you fight it.

A disorder called osteoporosis causes bones to deteriorate in the human body. When bones become less dense and thinner it is a result of osteoporosis. Bone fractures are far more common in those with osteoporosis.

Generally speaking, the bones in your body are dense and strong enough to support your weight and withstand most types of blows.

Your bones gradually lose part of their density and capacity to build up as you age. Your bones are weaker and considerably weaker than they should be if you have osteoporosis.

Most patients with osteoporosis are unaware of their condition until they have fractured bones.

Most parts of the bones might shatter with osteoporosis, however, the following are the most often affected when you have osteoporosis:

- hips (fractures of the hip)
- wrists
- spine (vertebral fractures)

Your chance of suffering from bone fractures decreases with the prompt diagnosis of osteoporosis by a medical professional.

See your doctor about having your bone density checked, particularly if you are older than 65, have experienced a bone fracture after the age of 50, or have osteoporosis in your biological family.

In the United States, according to research osteoporosis affects around 50 million individuals yearly who are above 50 years old.

According to experts, one in four persons designated male at birth over 50 and half of all people designated female are estimated to have osteoporosis.

Research also indicates that one in three persons over 50 who do not yet have osteoporosis also have osteopenia or a reduction in bone density.

Osteopenia patients have early indications of osteoporosis. Osteopenia can develop into osteoporosis if left untreated.

SYMPTOMS OF OSTEOPOROSIS:

Unlike many other medical disorders, osteoporosis does not exhibit symptoms. That's why medical professionals refer to it as a quiet illness occasionally.

You won't experience any symptoms or detect any changes that may indicate osteoporosis. You won't experience any symptoms of a medical condition such as a fever, headache, or stomachache.

The most frequent "symptom," which typically wouldn't affect you, is unexpectedly fracturing a bone, particularly if you have a minor fall or accident.

Although there are no obvious symptoms associated with osteoporosis, you may see some changes in your body that may indicate your bones are weakening or losing density. These cautionary indicators of osteoporosis may consist of the following:

- losing at least one inch off your height.
- alterations to your innate posture, such as stooping or leaning forward more.
- It shortens the breathing (if the compressed disks in your spine are causing your lung capacity to decrease).
- Lumbar spine discomfort, often known as lower back ache.

You may find it difficult to recognize changes in your physical appearance. Changes in your physique, particularly in your height or posture, maybe more noticeable to a loved one.

However, some people commonly joke that seniors are "shrinking," this might indicate that a senior should get tested for bone density.

CAUSES OF OSTEOPOROSIS:

As you age, your bones lose their capacity to repair and regenerate, which leads to osteoporosis.

Like every other part of your body, your bones are made of living tissue. Though it may not seem like it, throughout your life, they are always replenishing their cells and tissue.

Your body spontaneously replaces lost bone more often than not until about the age of thirty.

You gradually lose bone mass beyond the age of 35 because your body can no longer rebuild the broken bone as quickly.

Osteoporosis causes a faster loss of bone mass. Postmenopausal women experience an even greater loss of bone mass.

However, according to research, anyone can have osteoporosis. But some groups of people are likely to experience it. They include;

- an individual older than 50.
- Individuals classified as female at birth particularly those who are after menopause.
- Those with a family history of osteoporosis, if any member of your biological family is affected.
- those with "smaller frames" or those who are naturally slim Individuals with smaller statures may be more susceptible to bone loss since they often have lower natural bone density.

- those who consume tobacco a lot or smoke.

DISEASES OR ILLNESSES THAT CAN CAUSE OSTEOPOROSIS:

It is also important to note that some health conditions can cause one to develop osteoporosis, they include:

- Endocrine conditions include any illness that affects the thyroid, parathyroid glands, or hormones (e.g., diabetes, thyroid disease).
- disorders of the digestive system (such as inflammatory bowel disease [IBD] and celiac disease).
- bone-related autoimmune diseases (such as rheumatoid arthritis or ankylosing spondylitis, which is arthritis affecting the spine).
- Blood diseases (or blood-related malignancies, such as multiple myeloma).

It is important to keep in mind that the possibility of developing osteoporosis

may be increased by certain drugs or surgical procedures, which include:

- Diuretics are drugs that reduce blood pressure and help the body rid itself of excess fluid.
- corticosteroids, or anti-inflammatory drugs.
- drugs for the treatment of seizures.
- bariatric surgery, or losing weight.
- hormone therapy which is the treatment of cancer, particularly prostate and breast cancer.
- anticoagulants.
- Proton pump inhibitors (such as those used for acid reflux, which may impair the absorption of calcium in the body).

Osteoporosis might be more likely to occur if you follow certain food and exercise guidelines, such as:

- eating a diet deficient in calcium and vitamin D.
- insufficient exercise in physical terms.
- having more than two drinks of alcohol daily.

HOW TO MANAGE OR TREAT OSTEOPOROSIS:

The following are the various ways osteoporosis can be managed and treated:

- To strengthen the bone tissue you already have and slow down bone loss, your healthcare professional will recommend a treatment course.

Keeping bones from breaking is the most crucial aspect of treating osteoporosis.

- Exercises: You may strengthen your bones and all the tissue that is attached to them, such as your muscles, tendons, and ligaments, by engaging in regular exercise. Weight-bearing exercises may be recommended by your healthcare professional to build muscle and improve your balance.

Exercises that force your body to fight against gravity, such as tai chi, yoga, Pilates, and walking, can help you become more balanced and stronger without overstressing your bones.

It covers the exercises and motions that are best for you, you might need to consult with a physical therapist.

- Supplements for vitamins and minerals: You may require calcium

or vitamin D from your healthcare provider or prescription sources.

Your provider will determine your required medication's kind, quantity, and frequency.

OSTEOPOROSIS MEDICATION:

Your physician will advise you on the appropriate medications based on your individual needs.

Bisphosphonates and hormone therapy, such as replacement testosterone or estrogen, are among the most often prescribed drugs for osteoporosis.

Individuals who have a high risk of fractures or severe osteoporosis may require medicine, such as romosozumab, denosumab, and parathyroid hormone (PTH) analogs. Usually, injections are used to administer these drugs.

HOW TO PREVENT OR LOWER THE RISK OF OSTEOPOROSIS:

When you engage in routine exercises daily and ensure that you consume a lot of calcium and vitamin D in your daily meals you will be able to prevent osteoporosis.

It is very important to keep in mind that you should consult Your healthcare provider so he or she will be able to help you find several treatments that will be okay for you.

The following are different safety tips you should keep in mind to lower the risk of injury:

- Wear your seatbelt at all times.

- Wear the appropriate safety gear when participating in any sports and activities.
- Ensure that nothing might trip you or others in your house or business.
- When reaching for anything at home, always use the appropriate tools or equipment. Never stand on worktops, tables, or chairs.
- Adhere to a healthy workout and nutrition regimen.
- If you have trouble walking or are more likely to fall, use a cane or walker.

Please note that in all the chapters in this book, we are going to practice 40 different exercises for osteoporosis. These exercises will help to improve your general bone health, even if you are you are young or a senior. It will help to strengthen your body and prevent osteoporosis.

CHAPTER 2: EXERCISES TO IMPROVE BONE DENSITY AND FALL PREVENTION

The disorder known as osteoporosis makes bones brittle and feeble, increasing their vulnerability to fractures.

When the production of new bone does not keep up with the loss of existing bone, the illness develops. The hip, wrist, or spine are the most often fractured joints associated with osteoporosis.

It is very important to keep in mind that the bones support the body structure.

However, we are going to practice different exercises that can help to improve our bone density.

Note that before you perform any exercise in each chapter in this book ensure you do not have any kind of injury, but if you do, consult your health care provider and also ensure that you take a break if you feel tired when performing each round of the exercise.

The following are the exercises that can improve your bone density and prevent falls:

FOOT STOMPS EXERCISE:

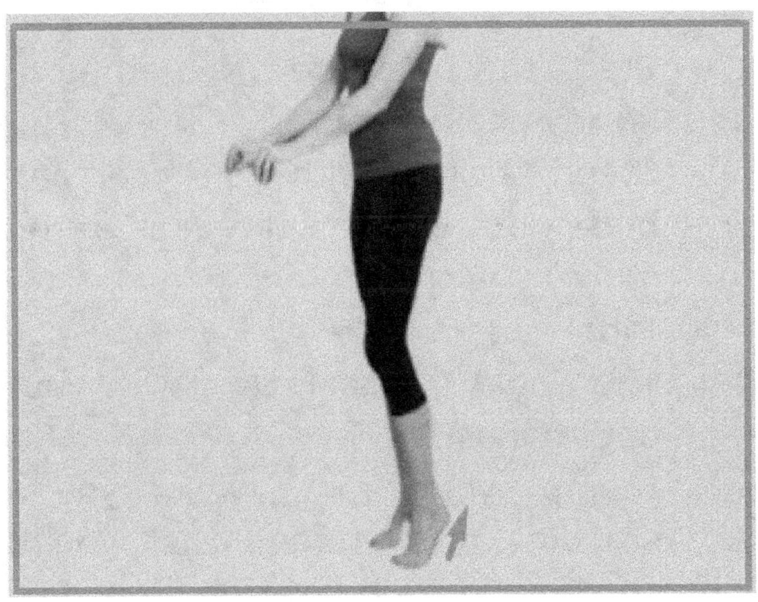

Engaging in physical activity such as foot stomps aimed at reducing osteoporosis involves targeting the major body parts that osteoporosis often affects, such as your hips. Stomping your feet is one activity that can help to strengthen the muscles and bones in your hips.

The following is the step-by-step guide for performing foot stomps:

- Start this exercise by getting a sturdy chair ready.
- Stand straight with your feet and hips-width apart at the back of the sturdy chair.
- Inhale and exhale.
- Then hold the chair firm with your both hands.
- Stomp your foot while you're standing and pretend that you're crushing a can beneath it.

- After four repetitions on one foot, switch to the other foot to complete the workout.
- If you get unsteady on your feet, grab a furniture or railing for support.

SHOULDER RAISES EXERCISE:

Lifting your shoulders requires the use of weights or a resistance band. Either standing or sitting can be used for this workout. This exercise helps to strengthen the bones around the shoulder region.

The following are the steps to perform this exercise:

- Pick up a dumbbell with both hands. Alternatively, grip an end in each hand and stomp on a resistance band.
- With your hands by your sides and your arms down, begin.

- Raise your arms straight out in front of you slowly, being careful not to lock your elbow.
- Raised to a level that is comfortable, but not higher than shoulder height.
- Do this eight or twelve times. Then you can take a break and repeat for a second set.

BICEP CURL EXERCISE:

You may use a resistance band or dumbbells ranging in weight from one to five pounds to do bicep curls exercise and also you can perform it either by standing or sitting, according to your comfort level.

The following are the guides to performing bicep curl:

- Hold a dumbbell in each hand. Alternatively, tread on a resistance band while keeping one end in each hand.

- Observe as the bicep muscles on the fronts of your upper arms tighten as you pull the bands or weights in toward your chest.
- To go back to where you were before, lower your arms.
- Observe eight to twelve times. If at all feasible, take a break and repeat for a second set.

HAMSTRING CURL:

Strengthen the muscles at the rear of your upper limbs with hamstring curls. This is an activity that you do while standing.

To help you balance better, you can put your hands on a substantial object or a piece of heavy furniture.

The following are steps to perform this exercise:

- Place your feet shoulder-width apart as you stand.
- Reposition your left foot such that only your toes will be in contact with the ground.
- To raise your left heel toward your buttocks, contract the muscles at the rear of your left leg.
- Return your left foot to its initial position with slow, deliberate movement.
- The exercise should be done eight to twelve times.
- After taking a break, repeat the exercise with your right leg.

SQUATS EXERCISE:

Squats are effective exercises for strengthening your buttocks and the front of your legs. This is not a deep squat exercise, but it can still be beneficial.

- Place your feet hip-width apart to begin. For balance, place your hands lightly on a strong counter or piece of furniture.
- lower yourself slowly then bend at the knees. Lean slightly forward while maintaining a straight back to feel the movement of your legs.
- Squat just as far as your thighs are from the floor.
- To get back to standing, tense your buttocks.
- Do this eight or twelve times over.

LEG RAISES WITH THE HIPS:

This exercise improves your balance and tones the muscles surrounding your hips. When you feel like you need to enhance your balance, put your hands on a substantial object like a piece of heavy furniture.

follow the steps below to perform the exercise:

- Place your feet hip-width apart to begin. Roll over onto your left foot.
- Raise your right foot to a maximum of 6 inches above the ground while maintaining a straight right leg.
- Bring your right leg down.
- Do the leg raise eight or twelve times then go back to where you were before and perform another set with your left leg.

SINGLE LEG STAND:

This exercise helps to improve balance in the body.

The following are the guides to performing this exercise:

- Get a sturdy chair
- Stand straight with your hands holding the back of the chair firm.

- Stand on one of your feet for at least a minute if you can, then alternate to the other feet.
- Try this at least 4 to 6 times if you can.

BALL SIT:

You can strengthen your abdominal muscles and improve your balance with this workout. It is best done with a big exercise ball.

Additionally, you can also get a "spotter" with you to assist you in keeping your balance.

The following are the steps to perform ball sit :

- With your feet flat on the ground, ensure you sit on the exercise ball.
- As you keep your equilibrium, try to keep your back as straight as you can.

- With your hands pointing forward, extend your arms out by your sides if you can.
- If at all feasible, maintain the posture for a full minute. Get up and take a break. You can do this exercise two more times if you can.

CHAPTER 3: SPINE STRENGTHENING EXERCISES FOR OSTEOPOROSIS

In this chapter, we are going to learn the various exercises that can help to strengthen the spine muscles. These exercises will also help the spine to stay stronger and prevent you from having osteoporosis.

To start each of these exercises Keep in mind to start with less resistance or make adjustments as necessary, breathe deeply during the exercises, and keep perfect form.

Before beginning any fitness program, it is essential to speak with a medical expert or physical therapist to be sure it is appropriate for you especially if you have any medical condition.

The following are the exercises that can help to strengthen your spine:

STANDING POSTURE ALIGNMENT:

Maintaining a good posture when standing eases the strain on your joints and spine, enhancing alignment and lowering the risk of compression fractures in your spinal bones.

However, for many other standing workouts, having proper alignment is a prerequisite.

Steps to perform the exercise:

- Position yourself so that you can stand comfortably, with your feet hip-width apart. If you feel that visual feedback is beneficial, you can utilize a mirror.
- Ensure that your spine is being drawn longer by a cord that is tugging you upward from the top of your head.

- At the same moment, see yourself rising taller while using your feet to push the floor away.
- Make sure your lower back is not arched as you gently push your shoulder blades together.
- Remember to engage your lower abdominal muscles.
- Maintain a straight posture and avoid overarching your lower back.
- Breathe regularly.
- Hold for a duration of 30 to 60 seconds then relax.

ABDOMINAL STRETCHING IN MANEUVER:

This is a fundamental core exercise that helps you build and engage the lower abdominal muscles which support your lower back is the abdominal drawing-in technique.

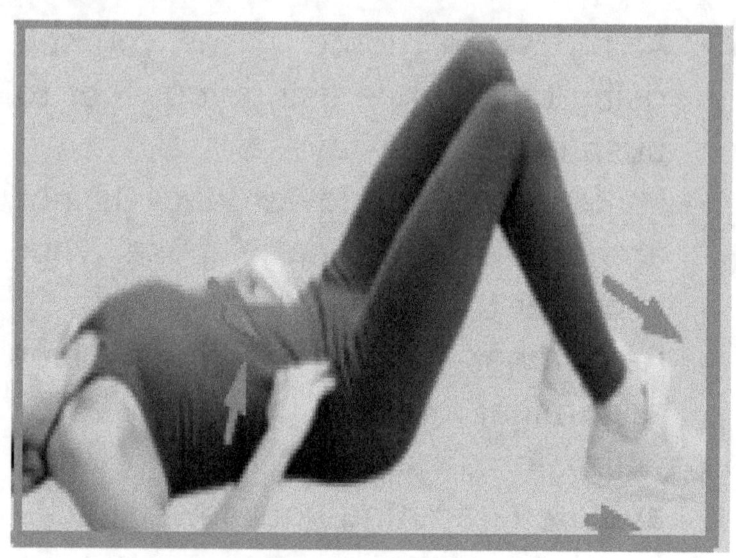

How to carry it out:

- With your feet level on the floor and your knees bent, start off reclining on a mat.
- To feel when your lower abdominal muscles are clenching, you can put your fingertips on the area directly inside your hip bones.
- Pulling your navel slowly toward your spine will help you tighten the muscles in your lower abdomen.

- As you tense your muscles, they should flatten toward the floor. They must not protrude.
- After ten seconds of holding the pose, release it.
- Don't hold back and breathe normally.
- Ten times over, repeat.

TAI CHI (THE GATHERING OF CHI):

A tai chi movement called gathering chi helps to warm up the muscles in your arms, shoulders, hips, knees, and middle of the back.

Being able to bear weight is crucial for maintaining the health of your spine, and it also promotes a better range of motion, which helps the body align and assume better posture throughout the day.

The following are the steps to take when you want to perform this exercise:

- To start tia chi you have to take a comfortable stand on your feet and ensure that your feet are placed hip-width apart.
- Make a circle with your hands up the sides of your body, and then gently let your palms drop. Picture yourself in the great outdoors, bathed in a soothing, colourful energy.
- Pull all that energy together and raise your arms in a circle above your head.
- Imagine that you are channelling that energy through each cell in your body as your palms go downward.
- As you gather your energy, softly bend your knees.
- Direct the energy through all of your organs, including your heart and lungs.
- Breathe regularly.

- Do this for about ten to twenty times.

ISOMETRIC THORACIC EXTENSION WHILE STANDING UP AGAINST A WALL:

The purpose of isometric thoracic extension, which involves standing against a wall, is to help develop and activate your thoracic spinal extensor muscles, which are the muscles that line each side of your spine.

This will help you maintain good posture and avoid slumping forward.

This is crucial for avoiding compression fractures and reducing the strain on your spine.

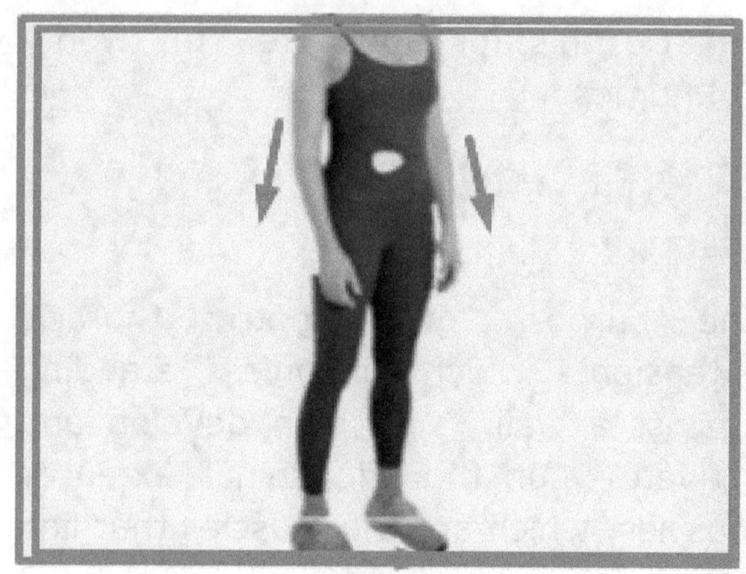

The following are the step-by-step instructions on how the perform this exercise effectively:

- Place your back against a wall to start.
- Your entire back should be flat against the wall while you stand with your feet approximately a foot apart from the wall and your knees slightly bent.

- As though attempting to arch your mid-back, gradually press your shoulders into the wall.
- You shouldn't shift or adjust your back position.
- Your midback muscles need to be tightened up.
- Take a few moments to hold this stance, then let go.
- Inhale regularly.
- Ten times, repeat.

STANDING HORIZONTALLY SHOULDER ABDUCTION WITH RESISTANCE BAND:

Resistance-based standing horizontal shoulder abduction strengthens the

shoulder and upper back muscles, which assist in maintaining proper posture and avoiding forward-rounded shoulders.

It incorporates an additional bone-building workout using a resistance band.

How to carry it out:

- Place your feet hip-width apart and stand tall.
- With both arms extended in front of you at a roughly 90-degree angle to your body, hold a resistance band. Face up with your palms facing up.
- Pull the band out to the sides with both arms while maintaining your arms straight and at chest level. Stop when your arms are in line with your shoulders. Then take a gradual step back to where you were before.
- Consider putting a pencil in the space between your shoulder blades.
- Breathe in a regular

SCAPULAR RETRACTION COMBINED WITH PRONE THORACIC EXTENSION:

While some people find it uncomfortable to lie on their stomach, doing a prone thoracic extension with scapular retraction is a fantastic way to strengthen your spine muscles. You may also perform this exercise on the floor with a pillow under your chest and belly.

Through the strengthening of the extensor muscles of the thoracic spine, this exercise helps lessen the strain on the spine and avoid a forward-slumped posture.

The following is how to carry out this exercise:

- Lay face down on a mat to start. If your lower back hurts in this posture, you can put foam or a pillow underneath your hips.

- Put both of your hands by your sides.
- Squeeze your shoulder blades together and raise your chest off the ground.
- After five to ten seconds, hold this posture, then return to the beginning position.
- Avoid lifting to the point that your lower back arches. Your midback's range of motion is the main target of this workout.
- Breathe regularly.
- Do two sets of five to ten repetitions each.

PRESSING THE NECK TOWARDS A RESISTANCE:

This workout is appropriate for all fitness levels. To carry it out:

- With a pillow underneath your head to maintain a neutral spine posture, lie on your back.
- For the spine to become longer and straighter, forcefully press the head down.
- Maintaining the head high, tuck the chin in without making any abrupt or jerky movements.
- After holding for a leisurely count of five, unwind for a short while.
- Till the muscles in your neck get fatigued, repeat ten times.
- Perform this workout every day in the morning and the evening. To advance, consider substituting a foam roller or rolled-up towel instead of a pillow.

CHEST LIFTS:

- Before beginning this workout, one should make sure they can easily lie on their stomach. To carry it out:
- If you're on the floor or a bed, lie on your stomach. It could be simpler to perform the workout with a pillow beneath the tummy.
- Maintaining a downward gaze, effortlessly raise the head and chest by drawing the shoulder blades together. Practice may be necessary since it may take some time to be able to raise the head or chest.
- After five seconds of holding, take a two-second break. Continue until you're exhausted.

SPINE STRENGTHENING EXERCISE:

This is a resistance band workout that combines bridges with chest openers. It enhances spinal stability and helps to strengthen the glutes and spine.

The steps to do this activity are as follows:

- lie on a mat and grasp a therapeutic band. Keep your feet flat on the ground, about two feet apart from your hips, and your hands shoulder-width apart.
- Squeeze your glute muscles while raising your hips toward the ceiling.
- Simultaneously spread your hands apart till they nearly touch the ground.

CHAPTER 4: OSTEOPOROSIS STRETCHES TO STRENGTHEN THE SHOULDER, NECK AND UPPER SPINE

It is important to keep in mind that stretching out tense muscles will always help to reduce pain and maintain proper posture and spinal mechanics.

However, in this chapter, we are going to be engaging in various stretches that will improve flexibility and reduce stiffness in the muscles.

The following are the stretches that improve flexibility:

STRENGTHENING OF THE EXTENSOR MUSCLES:

Complementing the spine's stabilizing function are the extensor muscles. To carry out this exercise the following are the steps to take:

- Strengthening of the extensor muscle
- Running parallel to the spine, the extensor muscles aid in its stability. To complete this task:
- Stand with your back against a wall, your spine straight, and proper posture.
- Position a bouncing ball between the upper back and the wall, gently pressing against it to keep it in place.
- Step back against the ball with your feet spread and away from the wall. While pivoting from the ankles, maintain a straight spine, hips, and knees.
- After holding for five seconds, take a two-second break.
- Continue until the muscles in your back or legs get fatigued.

- This is an exercise that people can perform every day, progressively increasing to 15–20 repetitions.

STRENGTHENING THE CALF

This exercise helps to strengthen the calf.

- To perform this stretch, stand and hold a table or chair for support.
- Retrace your right leg step.
- Bend your left knee forward gently.
- Verify that the back is straight and that both feet' heels are on the ground. The right calf should be stretched in the back.
- After 15 seconds of holding, switch to the other leg.

ACROSS-THE-CHEST STRETCH:

Your shoulder joint and the surrounding muscles will become more flexible and have a wider range of motion after performing this exercise.

If you have shoulder soreness during this exercise, drop your arm.

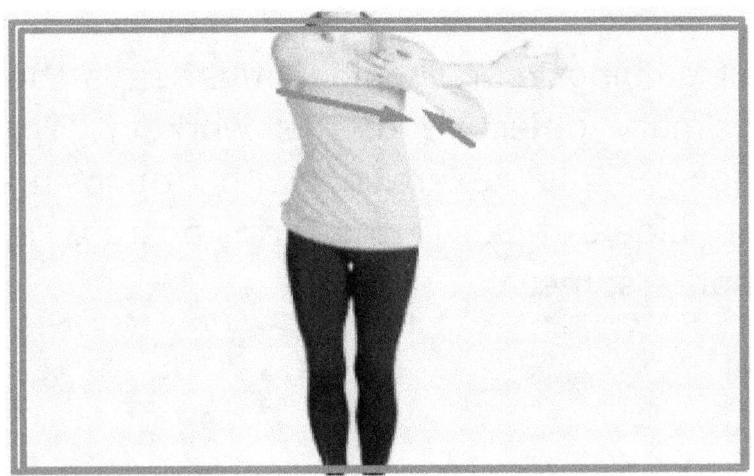

To start this stretch the following are the various steps to take:

- Firstly stand straight.
- Move your right arm over your chest.
- Either place it in the bend of your left elbow or support your arm with your left hand.

- For as long as a minute, maintain this posture.
- On the other side, repeat.
- Repeat 3-5 times on each side.

SPINAL ROLLS AND EAGLE ARMS:

Stretching your shoulder muscles is the primary objective of this workout. Try doing this exercise with opposing shoulders held if the arm posture is bothersome.

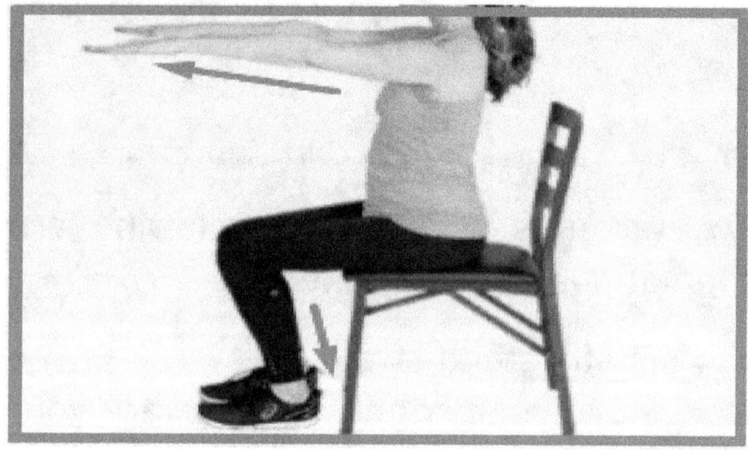

The following are the guides to performing this exercise

- To start this workout, sit on a chair and spread your arms apart.
- Your right arm should be on top when you cross your elbows in front of your torso.
- Make sure your hands and forearms are together by bending your elbows.
- Put your palms together with your right hand by reaching around.
- For fifteen seconds, stay in this posture.
- Draw your elbows in toward your chest and twist your spine while exhaling.
- Spread your ribs and raise your arms as you inhale.
- After a minute, keep up this motion.
- Repeat on the other side.

this exercise helps to strengthen the neck and shoulder muscles Throughout this exercise, keep your hips pointing forward. Permit your lower back to begin to twist.

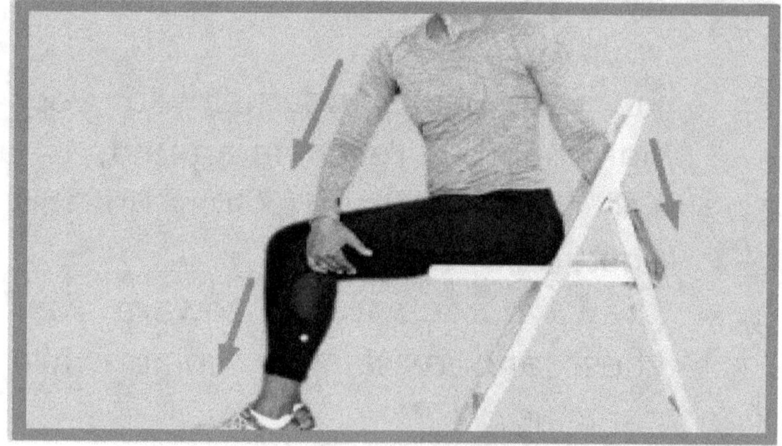

- Place your ankles exactly beneath your knees while seated on a chair.
- Bring the back of your left hand up to your thigh by rotating your upper body to the right.
- Put your right hand down where it feels comfortable.

- Maintain this posture for a maximum of thirty seconds.
- Do the same on the left side.
- Repeat three to five times on each side.

SHOULDERS CIRCLE:

You can increase flexibility and warm up your shoulder joints with this workout. The following are the guides to performing this exercise:

- Place your left hand behind a chair while you stand there.
- Let your right-hand dangle downward.
- Make five circles with your right hand in each direction.
- On the other side, repeat.
- Repeat two to three times a day.

INFANT POSE:

This exercise helps your neck, shoulders, and back to all feel less tense in this restorative position. Please note that for support, place a pillow beneath your knees, forehead, or chest.

The following are the various steps to take when performing this exercise:

- Bring your knees slightly wider than your hips and your big toes together in Downward Dog Pose.
- Lean your hips back into your heels and raise your arms above your head.
- Let your shoulders and spine relax as you let your chest drop heavily to the ground.
- For a maximum of five minutes, hold this stance.

PUT THE NEEDLE IN THE THREAD EXERCISE:

Your upper back, shoulders, and chest will all feel less tense after doing this exercise. To provide support, ensure you place a pillow or block beneath your head or shoulder then proceed with the steps below:

- Take a kneeling position to begin. Raise your right hand, palm out from your body, and point it toward the ceiling.
- With your palm facing up, lowering your arm will bring it beneath your chest and to the left side of the body.
- To prevent falling into this location, engage your right shoulder and arm.
- For stability, keep your left hand on the ground, raise it to the sky, or bring it around to the inner of your right thigh.
- For a maximum of 30 seconds, maintain this posture.
- Before resuming this stretch, unwind in Child's Pose.

DOORWAY SHOULDER WORKOUT:

This exercise strengthens the shoulders and expands your chest.

The following the steps to perform this exercise:

- Make a 90-degree angle with your arms and elbows while you stand in a doorway.
- Press your palms onto the door frame's sides and step your right foot forward.
- Lie forward and contract your abs. As long as 30 seconds, maintain this posture.
- Stretch again by placing your left foot forward.
- Repeat each side three times.

DOG POSE DOWNWARD:

Your back and shoulder muscles are stretched and strengthened by this inversion posture.

Follow the steps below so you can effectively do the exercise:

- Get on your hands and knees to begin. Raise your hips toward the ceiling by applying pressure with your hands.
- When you equally distribute your weight into your hands and feet, keep your knees slightly bent.
- Bring your head toward your feet to bend your shoulders overhead while maintaining a straight spine.
- Take a minute or so to maintain this stance.

RELEASE OF THE NECK EXERCISE:

You may gently release tension in your shoulders and neck by performing this exercise.

Follow the steps below to perform the exercise:

- Raise your chin close to your chest. you are going to be experiencing stretch around the back of your neck.
- To extend your right shoulder, gently tilt your head to the opposite side of your shoulder.
- maintain this posture for at least a minute.
- On the other side, repeat.
- Repeat 3-5 times on each side.

CHAPTER 5: OSTEOPOROSIS STRETCHES FOR STRENGTH AND FULL BODY BALANCE

In this chapter, we are going to dive into different exercises that will help to improve the body balance, and posture and strengthen the muscles.

It is important to keep in mind that these workouts are specifically designed to heal osteoporosis thereby strengthening the muscles and leading to better posture and improving balance.

The following are the exercises that can help to strengthen the muscles, and improve balance and posture:

CHAIR SQUAT:

This is an excellent strengthening and balance workout for the entire body. You can use a chair or a sofa depending on which is your choice. It's better if the chair has an armrest so you can support yourself by resting your fingertips on it.

The instructions to follow when performing this exercise are:

- In front of a chair, stand with your feet wider than shoulder-width apart. Lean forward, lengthen your spine, and roll your shoulders back.
- Lower your body, flex your knees, and push your hips back.
- After giving the chair a tap, rise back to your starting position.
- Repeat ten times, increasing the number of repetitions and sets.

Note that you should avoid doing this exercise if you are suffering from health conditions such as arthritis of the knee and lower back aches.

CHAIR CALF RAISES EXERCISE:

This exercise helps to strengthen the calf muscles.

The following are the actions to take when performing this exercise

- Put your hands on the backrest of a chair as you stand behind it. Look forward while rolling your shoulders back. This is where everything begins.
- Take off your heels from the floor.
- After 5-8 seconds of pausing, release the air and plant your heels on the floor.
- Repeat fifteen times.

LEG SWING BALANCE EXERCISE:

This is another activity that helps improve balance and is beneficial for both individuals who already have osteoporosis and those who wish to reduce their risk. For this workout, you will need a chair for support.

The following the the steps to take when performing this exercise.

- Holding the backrest with your right hand, take a seat to your right. Roll your shoulders back while standing with your feet hip-width apart.
- Raise and extend your left foot laterally off the ground. Point your toes forward at all times.
- Bring your leg over the front of your right leg by swinging it back.
- Repeat ten times, then switch to your right leg.
- Take a position behind the chair. Put your hands on the backrest, one or both.
- Raise your right leg off the ground and do a back-and-forth swing.

- Ten times over, repeat the same steps for the left leg.

BICEP CURLS USING RESISTANCE BANDS:

As you age, your hand bones weaken as well, particularly the wrists.

Engaging in weighted osteoporosis activities, like working with a resistance band, enhances hand muscle strength and flexibility, which in turn promotes better bone health. A flat, open-ended therapeutic band is required.

The following are the steps to do this activity:

- Put your right foot on one end of the resistance band.
- Stretching out your arms, grasp the opposite end with your right hand.

- Keep your elbow pulled up against your body as you curl up your hand.
- Return your hand to its initial position.
- Before changing hands, repeat this ten times.

TRUNK ROTATION EXERCISE:

This is a low-impact exercise that improves spine strength.

Follow the actions below to perform this exercise:

- Start this exercise by placing your feet hip-width apart as you stand.
- Place your arms across each other on your chest to form an X letter.
- Look forward while repositioning your shoulders. This is where everything begins.
- Rotate your upper torso in both directions.

- Repeat fifteen times.

LYING LEG DROPS EXERCISE:

For those who have osteoporosis, this is a low-impact workout that strengthens the core. To support your lower back, use a rolled towel.

The steps to performing this exercise are:

- On a mat, arrange a rolled towel.
- Carefully lay down on the mat. Place the rolled towel exactly where the curvature of your lower back occurs.
- Raise both of your legs off the ground, maintaining a 90-degree angle with your knees bent. This is where everything begins.
- Lower your right leg.
- Raise your right leg back to the beginning position after tapping the ground.

- To finish one rep, repeat the identical movement with your left leg.
- Repeat fifteen times.

CORE-STRENGTHENING EXERCISE:

Once you can perform leg drops without discomfort, consider strengthening your spine with weighted exercises. For this workout, you'll need a thin, open-ended resistance band.

The following are the guides to do this exercise effectively:

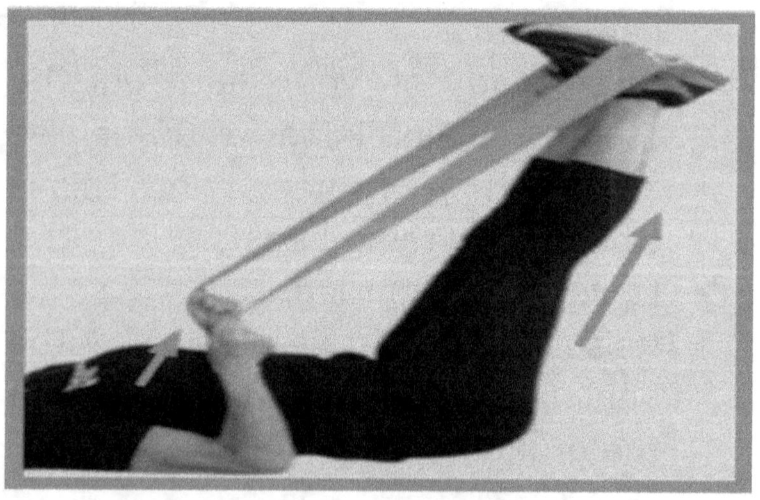

- Start this exercise by gently lying on a mat and grasping a resistance band as you can see in the picture above.
- Wrap your feet in the band. Maintain your legs stretched and perpendicular to the floor while holding onto the band's end. This is where everything begins.
- Bring your knees up to your chest and flex them.
- Return to the beginning posture by pushing your legs up.
- Repeat ten to fifteen times.

CHAPTER 6: PILATES STRETCHES TO IMPROVE FLEXIBILITY

It is important to keep in mind that Pilate activities are very good for preventing or curing osteoporosis.

Pilate exercises help to strengthen the core, increase bone density, increase muscle mass and keep the body flexible and balanced.

However, in this chapter, we are going to do some pilates that will help us to improve flexibility and prevent the bones and muscles from getting stiff.

The following are the different pilates for flexibility:

HIP STRENGTHENING STRETCH:

Exercise like this lowers the chance of hip fractures and osteoporosis. To do it, you'll need a loop resistance band.

The following are the guides to performing this exercise:

- Take a seat on a mat. Adhere to a resistance band in a loop just above the knee.
- Lay on your right side, rest your left hand on the mat, and use your right hand to support your head.
- As seen in the illustration, maintain a 90-degree angle between your thighs and your shin.
- Raise your right leg toward the sky. Don't make it longer.
- Take it down.
- Before swapping sides, repeat this ten times.

This exercise helps to strengthen the body.

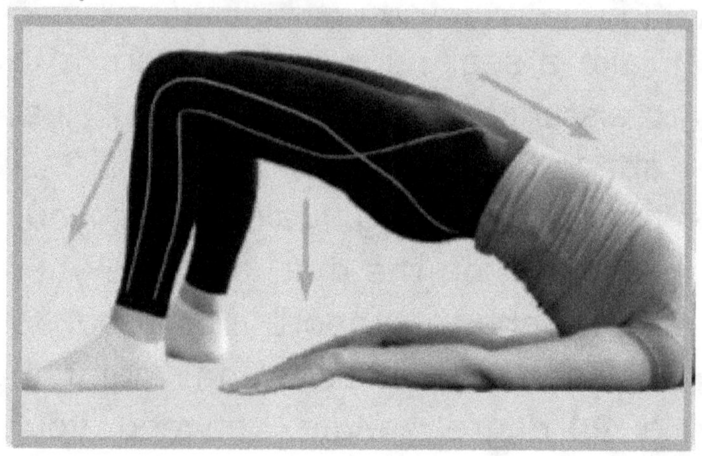

- Lay flat on your back on a yoga mat or any other comfortable surface.
- With your knees bent and your arms at your sides, position your feet flat on the floor, hip-width apart.
- Inhale and contract your abdominal muscles.

- Lift your hips toward the ceiling while applying pressure through your heels and squeezing your glutes.
- When you reach the peak of the bridge posture, form a straight line with your shoulders and knees.
- As you maintain your core muscles contracted, hold the bridge posture for a few seconds.
- Breathe out as you slowly return your hips to the beginning position.
- Repeat this for two to three sets of ten to fifteen reps.

SIDEKICK PILATE:

This pilate helps to strengthen the lower parts of the body such as the abdominal, flexors, and hip extensors.

The following are the guides to performing this pilate:

- With your lower arm extended above and your ear resting on it, lie on your side. Your legs should be angled between 30 and 45 degrees in front of your torso as you move your feet forward and maintain straight knees.
- Consider pulling on a belt a little bit to raise and sculpt your abs.
- Raise your front leg till it is parallel to your hip.
- Breathe in to propel your leg forward without hunching over or bending your back.
- Kick your leg back with an exhale, expanding your hip and using your hamstrings and glutes.
- Aim to maintain a long spine and stacked hips throughout the whole range of motion of your leg, without tucking, rolling, or arching your pelvis.
- After 8–10 repetitions, alternate.

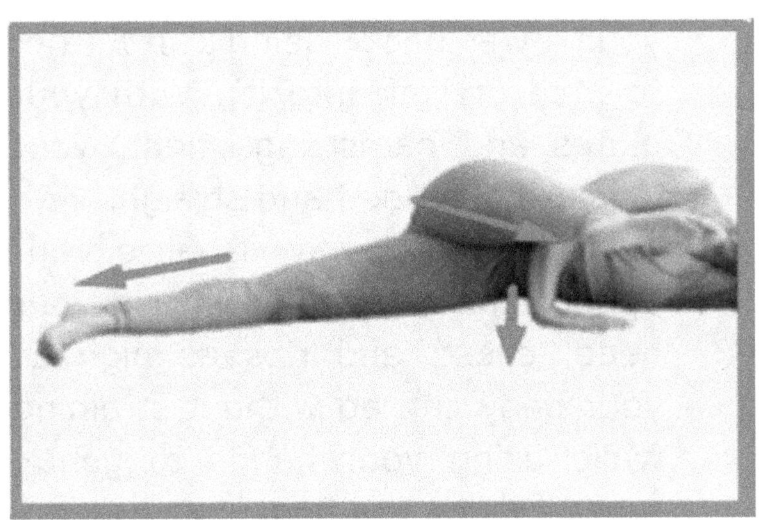

SWAN DIVE PILATE:

This pilate helps to strengthen the spine, abdominal muscles and the hips:

The following are how to do this pilate effectively:

- Place your hands flat on the floor, parallel to your shoulders, and lie face down on the floor with your elbows bent.
- Start by tensing your body, pulling your abs in and up, and extending

your lower back (being careful not to arch or sink into it). With your glutes and hamstrings tight, your legs are extended and straight.

- Take a breath and visualize your upper head extending out. Lift your head, chest, and ribs as high as your body can go without straining while using your hands to gently press against the floor.
- Return to the mat by extending your torso with an exhale.
- Five to eight times, repeat.

BIRD DOG PILATE:

This exercise helps to strengthen the lower parts of the body and spine.

Follow the step-by-step guide do the pilate:

- With your hands behind your shoulders and your knees beneath your hips, begin on all fours.

- Try to keep your head in alignment with your shoulders and maintain a neutral spine.
- Draw your abdominals in and up by exhaling. Lift one leg behind you and the opposing arm in front, without changing your weight or arching your back.
- Take a breath, and hold the pose for three slow counts.
- Take a controlled breath to lower your hand and leg back to the ground.
- Continue on the opposite side.